BALANCED FOOD

— for —

BETTER HEALTH

Based on Food Security and Biotechnology

DR. PRAKASH BHARODIA
& SNEHAL PATEL, MS

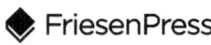 FriesenPress

Suite 300 - 990 Fort St
Victoria, BC, V8V 3K2
Canada

www.friesenpress.com

Copyright © 2021 by Dr. Prakash Bharodia and Snehal Patel
First Edition — 2021

ISBN
978-1-5255-5731-6 (Hardcover)
978-1-5255-5732-3 (Paperback)
978-1-5255-5733-0 (eBook)

1. Health & Fitness, Nutrition

Distributed to the trade by The Ingram Book Company

This book is dedicated to
Dr. Bharodia's mother and father,
Nanduben and Shamjibhai Bharodia

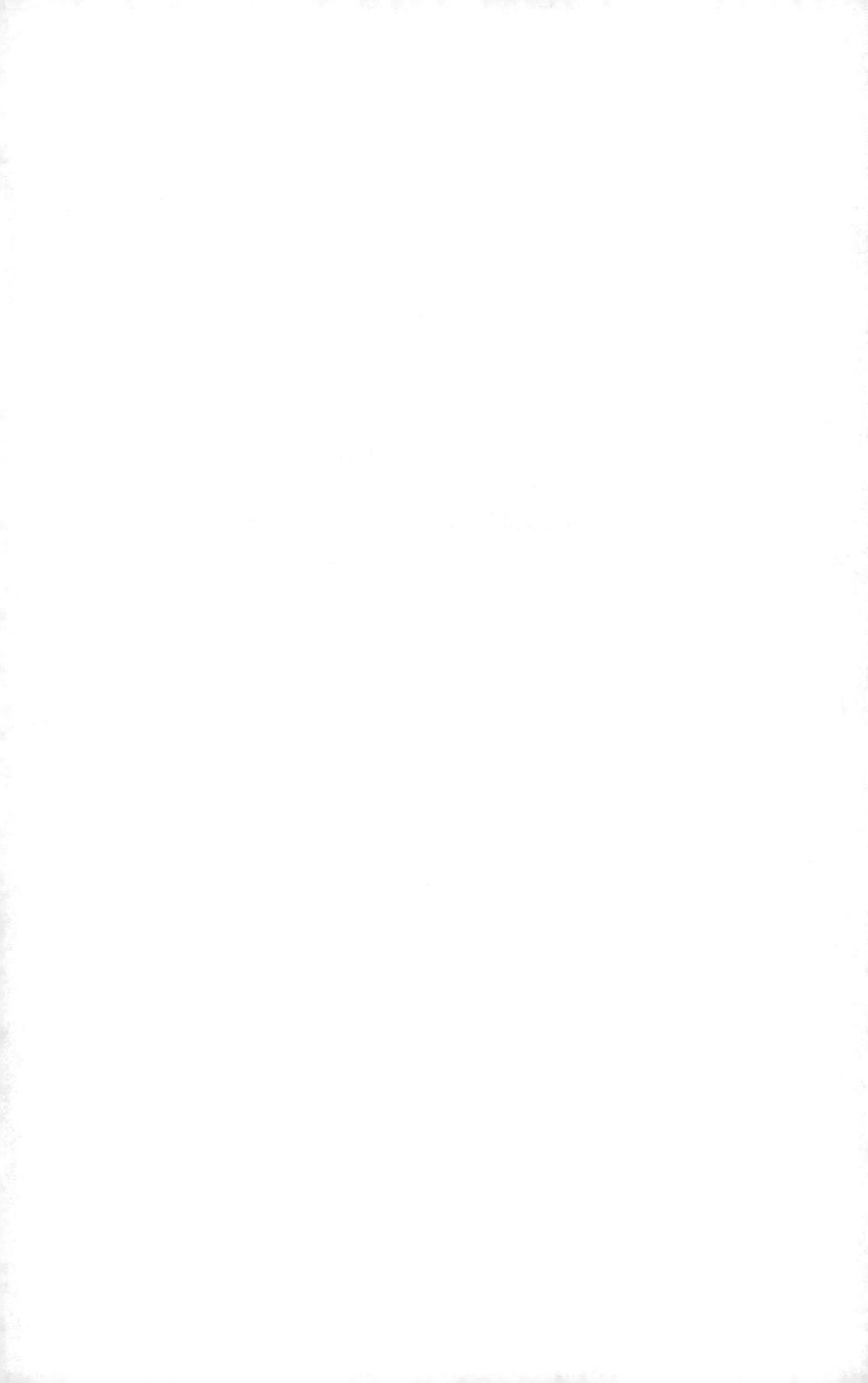

Acknowledgements

We wish to express our sincere thanks to the friends and associates who have helped us during the preparation of this book, particularly Dr. R.M. Shah, Dr. M.S. Basu, Dr. P.S. Reddy, Dr. H.R. Kher, Dr. P.M. Vaghasia, Dr. G. Nagarjan, Dr. K.B. Saxena, and Dr. Laxaman Singh.

We also thank Gujarat Agricultural University, the Directorate of Oilseeds Research, the National Research Centre for Groundnut, the International Crop Research Institute of Semiarid Tropics, the International Research Institute of Wheat and Maize, Gujarat Ayurvedic University, the Food Technology Institute, and the Central Institute of Medical and Aromatic Plants for providing necessary facilities.

We will never forget the healthy help and encouragement of Dr. Bharodia's wife Bharti, son Mayur, and daughters Snehal and Hemal as well as daughter-in-law Sweta and sons-in-law Manish and Birju during the preparation of this book.

We are also very thankful to the publisher, book sellers, and advertising media, who have made considerable effort in promoting this book to readers.

CONTENTS

PREFACE

THIS BOOK HAS BEEN WRITTEN with the idea of providing necessary information about balanced foods for the better health and strength of the body. The diets mentioned are not medical prescriptions or advice but simply guidelines and general recommendations, which have been generated through the course of food-research and health findings about herbs. We know that in their daily diets people regularly take in all the nutritional components of foods like carbohydrates, proteins, fats, vitamins, minerals, and roughage. To obtain this nutrition they consume plant-based foods like cereal, legumes, oils, spices, fruits, vegetables as well as animal-products like milk and milk products, meat, eggs, fish, etc. But in order to balance the nutrients in our bodies for better health and strength, it is important to know what kinds of foods we should eat and how much should be consumed in our daily dietary schedules.

Foods contain differing amounts of nutritional components. Therefore, we have broken down this information into simple categories so that people of all ages can understand very easily. Moreover, if people follow this food schedule from childhood there will be less susceptibility to various diseases and disorders throughout their lives. But even if people don't begin following these suggestions until later in life, they can avoid many diseases and disorders at later life stages, as well cure existing diseases and disorders from which they may already be suffering.

We also provide information about anti-aging nutrients and foods, which help to slow down the aging process for youthful looks and better sexual performance.

Brief information about foods and nutrients that help to improve appearance is also included here, separately.

The weekly schedule of nutrients and foods for maintaining healthier, fitter bodies will be helpful to everyone. However, individual growth, weight, and energy needs must be taken into consideration. For instance, young people require more food than older people do. Something that must also be taken into consideration is how long each nutrient is retained in the body and remains effective. Nutrients like carbohydrates, proteins, and fats are stored and retained longer in the body while nutrients like vitamins and minerals remain in the body for a shorter time.

We have taken into consideration the seasonal availability of different foods and materials, vegetarian and non-vegetarian choices, and the human tendency toward diversification in selection of foods. Diseases and disorders have also been considered, and we have suggested more than one food or nutritional count for each of the food regimens.

There is information on herbal cures, medicinal foods, and drugs that substitute for foods/nutrients. We also discuss how more nutrients are retained in foods and which foods are the most useful for household purposes.

I, Dr. Bharodia have worked as a research scientist on food crops like cereal, legumes, oilseeds, etc., and I am a professor of post-graduate study in genetic engineering and biotechnology.

I have combined my knowledge of the biochemical properties of crops with the nutritional quality of foods for better health. During my research I have bred and developed many high-yielding and better-quality varieties of different crops, which have helped to solve certain food shortages. That gave me the idea to write this book, in order to help people minimize their health problems by eating natural foods.

My daughter, Snehal Patel, has a master's degree in Plant Science and Genetics and she contributed equally to the preparation of this book.

At present, plenty of information is available about nutrients, foods, and health, but few people are actually using it in their daily lives, either because they don't think seriously about their future health or because they feel the practical implementation of better nutrition would be too complicated. That's why we have prepared this book in an extremely short, simple format that everyone can understand and employ very easily in their lives.

We wish everyone health, happiness, and long life.

Dr. Prakash Bhardoia
PhD (Plant Science and Genetics)

Snehal Patel MS
(Plant Science and Genetics)

I. NUTRITIONAL FOOD COMPONENTS

IN THE FIELD OF AGRICULTURAL PRODUCTION, an application of biotechnological achievements like biogenic crop varieties, biofertilizers, and biopesticides is helping to reduce water, air, and soil pollution along with increasing the production of higher-quality food crops for better food security. Food security does not refer only to food supply but to nutritional balance for health and strength. Plant-based foods include grain cereals, legumes, oils, spices, dried fruits, fruits, and vegetables. Animal resources consist of milk and other dairy products, meat, eggs, fish, etc. Therefore, foods are classified into two categories as per people's dietary habits: vegetarian food, which is derived from plant-based food and dairy products; and non-vegetarian food, from animal products like meat, eggs, fish, etc. It is the duty and the responsibility of governments of different countries to meet food security needs by supplying sufficiently balanced food materials, either by producing in their own countries or by importing from others.

In food security, balanced nutrition means the availability of food that supplies necessary absorbable nutritional components like carbohydrates, protein, fat, roughage, vitamins, minerals, water, etc. appropriate for people's ages and body weights. Food nutrients generate biological energy called calories, which are required for the proper functioning of bio-physio processes within the body. As a result, body growth and vigor are maintained properly, and such healthy bodies can work efficiently. Food nutrients are of two types: macronutrients like carbohydrates, proteins, and fats, which are required in large quantity because they generate energy. Then there are micronutrients like vitamins and minerals, which are required in small quantity because they don't create energy but only help in the release of energy from macronutrients. Here is how our body is built up of different components: water (60%), protein (17%), fat (15%), minerals (5%), carbohydrates (1%) and nuclei (4%).

(1) CARBOHYDRATES

Carbohydrates are the most important energy-generating components and are present in almost all foods. Carbohydrates like starch and sugar, which are converted in glucose, are known as blood sugar and they provide essential energy to the body— one gram of carbohydrate gives four calories of energy. Being a working energy components, carbohydrates are required in large quantity as compared to other food components. About 150 to 200 gm. of carbohydrates are required per person per day to generate enough energy for proper functioning of the body. If more carbohydrates are taken in, then they are stored in the form of glucose or glycogen in the liver or in the muscles as fat. When the body requires more fuel, then this fat is again converted to glucose. All the cereal foods, such as wheat, oat, barley, rice, maize, millet, sorghum, etc. are rich in carbohydrate content (85-90%) and often make up the major part of our daily diets. These cereals are used as flour or whole grain in many of the cuisines of the world.

Grain Cereals as a Source of Carbohydrates in Foods:

Wheat is the most important staple food crop in almost all the countries of the world. Wheat grains contain about 85% carbohydrates and 13% protein. Generally, wheat flour without fiber, called white-flour, is used in bakeries for making foods like bread, biscuits, cake, cookies, noodles, pasta, pizza, etc. Nowadays, since the importance of fiber in food is understood, wheat flour is used in making various types of multigrain breads. These whole-grain breads contain vitamins like thiamine, niacin, riboflavin, folate, pantothenic acid, and vitamin E. Whole-grain breads are more nutritious because they contain balanced nutrients like carbohydrates, proteins, fats, vitamins, minerals, roughage, and water. Wheat is the main source of carbohydrates in most human diets. However, it is low in lysine, protein, and fat. Therefore, wheat flour is often mixed with 10% maize flour and 5% soybean flour to make it a nutritionally balanced food. This multigrain flour contains a balanced amount of all the food components like carbohydrates, protein, fat, vitamins, minerals, and roughage.

Rice is the important staple food after wheat in the Asian, African, and Arabian countries of the world. Rice grains contain about 87% carbohydrates and 11% protein.

Rice is consumed as whole grain after steaming or boiling and is served with vegetables and/or fish or meat. Rice flour is also used in many food preparations. Rice is rich in carbohydrates, and so, for balance, it is best eaten with protein-rich foods like meat, yogurt, chicken, fish, etc.

Maize ranks third in importance of the cereal foods. It is generally grown for food and fodder in almost all the countries of the world. Maize kernels contain about 88% carbohydrates and 10% protein. Maize flour is used in multigrain breads, brans, and many other food preparations. The green kernels of sweet corn maize can be eaten after steaming or in soup. The matured and dried kernels of maize are used for making popcorn. Maize flour is often mixed with soybean and grain-legume flour for making breads and for other food preparations. Likewise, maize bran is eaten with milk or grain legumes.

Pearl Millet is also an important cereal food crop in some countries like India, Africa, and the United States. Millet is also grown for fodder purposes.

The grains or seeds of millet are small and contain about 73% carbohydrate and 15% protein. Millet flour is used in baking and can be steamed as a whole grain. Though low in protein, millet contains high amounts of iron.

Sorghum is considered a minor grain crop and is grown for food and fodder purposes in countries like India, Africa, etc. Sorghum flour contains about 87% carbohydrates and 12% protein. The flour is used in baking and other food preparations in tribal areas.

Don't forget your carbohydrates ...

(2) PROTEIN

Protein is the most important component of food. It is required for physical and mental growth, vigor, and the development of the human body. Thus it is called the building-block food for the human body. Protein is available from both plant and animal sources.

Protein is of two types. One is called complete protein and has the proper balance of all eight amino acids. It is found in foods of animal origin like milk and milk products, meat, eggs, fish, seafood, etc. The second is incomplete protein and does not have the proper balance of all eight essential amino acids. It is found in the plant-based proteins of legumes, nuts, beans, grains, seeds, etc.

Protein of animal origin is completely digestible and is more efficiently used by the body. Protein of plant origin is not completely digestible and is less efficiently used. That's why both types of proteins should be taken in combination. For example, rice and beans can be eaten with either yogurt or cheese.

Amino acids are the building blocks of protein. There are twenty-two amino acids in total and they are required for protein synthesis. Eight of them are essential amino acids like leucine, isoleucine, lysine, methionine, phenylalanine, threonine, tryptophan, and valine, which are not synthesized in the body and are provided through foods. The ninth essential amino acid is histidine, which is required for infants and children.

Generally, for normal growth and strength, people require fifty grams of protein each day. However, those people who eat grain cereals daily will only need twenty-five grams of protein from either grain legumes or meat. The grain cereals can contribute the remaining twenty-five grams of protein. Protein gives four calories of energy per gram of consumption.

Grain legumes like chickpeas, peas, soybeans, beans, moong (green gram) beans, black lentils, pigeon peas, black-eyed (goat) peas, and groundnuts, etc. contain about 23% protein. Grain legumes are the main source of protein in vegetarian diets while dairy products are a secondary source.

In non-vegetarian diets, animal products like meat, eggs, fish, etc. are the main source of protein.

Plant and Animal Sources of Protein in Food:

Grain legumes are eaten in the form of whole grains or split grains, as flour, and as green seeds/pods.

The seed coat of grain legumes contains anti-nutritional substances and can cause flatulence. They should be soaked in warm or room-temperature water overnight. In the morning, the water should be drained and the grains rinsed with clean water two to three times. Once all the anti-nutritional substances are washed from the seed coat, then the legumes can be cooked in boiling water or steamed until they become soft. Half frying in oil and adding some salt and spices should make them delicious. Eat them with either rice or bread.

The immature and green seeds of legumes like peas, pigeon peas, black-eyed peas, beans, lentils, chickpeas, etc. are used as vegetables. The green seeds are more nutritious and digestible than matured seeds. Foods prepared with green grain legumes are delicious and contain more protein, vitamins, and minerals.

The flour of grain legumes like chickpeas, soybeans, mung beans, etc. is used for making different breakfast and children's foods.

Nutritional components in green seeds of different legumes

Nutritional components	Green Legumes			
	Peas	Pigeon peas	Beans	Chick-peas
Moisture (%)	72.1	66.1	70.1	78.5
Carbohydrate (%)	15.9	18.9	14.5	16.7

Protein (%)	7.2	9.8	8.2	8.1
Fat (%)	0.1	1.0	0.7	0.6
Mineral (mg/100 gram)				
Calcium	20.0	27.0	25.0	18.0
Magnesium	34.0	59.0	42.0	50.0
Copper	0.2	0.1	0.2	0.1
Iron	1.5	1.1	1.4	1.2
Vitamins (mg/100 gm)				
A. Carotene	63.0	469.0	75.0	85.0
B1- Thiamin	0.1	0.3	0.1	0.2
B2- Riboflavin	0.01	0.3	0.2	0.1
B3- Niacin	0.8	3.0	2.5	2.0
D. Hydro cholesterol	0.0	20.0	8.0	9.0

Milk and Milk Products as Sources of Protein in Foods:

Among the various animal food products, milk is the best source of protein. It is consumed by vegetarians and non-vegetarians alike. The milk of cows, buffalos, goats, sheep, camels, etc. contains about 3.5 to 4.5% protein, which is easily digested by infants, and young and old people. Moreover, milk and milk food products like milk powder, yogurt, cheese, chocolate, butter, cream, etc. are available in almost all the countries of the world. Milk also contains essential minerals like Ca, P, K, Mg, Na, Fe and vitamins A, B complex and C in various amounts.

Nutritional Components in Milk

Nutritional components	Milk			
	Cow	Buffalo	Goat	Sheep
Water (%)	87.5	82.0	86.8	85.2
Carbohydrate (%)	4.4	5.0	4.6	4.2
Protein (%)	3.2	4.3	3.2	3.5
Fat (%)	4.4	6.5	4.5	4.7
Calories	67	117	67	71
Mineral (mg/100 gm)				
Calcium	100	210	170	181
Potassium	140	90	110	107
Phosphorus	70	130	110	109
Sodium	74	170	110	112
Faric	2	0.2	0.3	0.3
Vitamins (mg/100 gm)				
Vitamin A	52	48	55	52
B1 Thymine	0.05	0.04	0.05	0.04
B2 Riboflavin	0.49	0.1	0.04	0.06
B3 Niacin	8.10	0.1	0.3	0.5
B9 Folic Acid	8.50	5.6	1.3	1.4
Vitamin C	2.0	1.0	1.0	1.1

Don't forget your protein ...

(3) FATS

Fat is also a most important component of our daily foods. It gives more energy (9 calories/gm) as compared to carbohydrates or protein (4 calories/gm). Generally, fifty grams of fat is required per day in our daily food for maintaining the energy level for better health and strength.

Fats are available from plant sources (referred to as oils) and from animal sources (referred to as fat). Both contain different fatty acids, which determine the nutritional quality of oils and fats. Dietary fat or food fats are biochemically known as triglycerides, every molecule of fat having one molecule of glycerol and three molecules of fatty acids.

The fatty acids are of two types; one is saturated and the second is unsaturated. Further, the unsaturated fatty acids are of two types; one is monounsaturated fatty acid (MUFA) and the second is polyunsaturated fatty acid (PUFA). Higher consumption of saturated fat increases the LDL (Low Density Lipoprotein), which increases the level of cholesterol in blood and can cause heart disease. The consumption of unsaturated fat, either MUFA or PUFA, increases the level of HDL (High Density Lipoprotein). This lowers the level of cholesterol in the blood and reduces the possibility of heart disease. Lipoprotein is composed of protein and fat. It works as a carrier of cholesterol in blood vessels. Consequently, dietary fats have a direct relationship to the level of cholesterol in the blood.

Lipoprotein is composed of protein and fat. It works as a carrier of cholesterol in blood vessels. So the difference in the behavior of the cholesterol depends upon the protein to which it is bound. LDL carries 65% blood cholesterol and VLDL carries 15%. This can block arteries and increase the chance of heart disease. On the other hand, HDL carries 20% blood cholesterol and is mainly composed of lecithin. Therefore, it breaks plaque and transports cholesterol without blocking/clogging arteries.

People with big hips and trim waists tend to have higher levels of HDL as compared to those with potbellies. Blood cholesterol tests also measure levels of triglycerides. They are different from cholesterol, but there is a relationship between them. Though triglyceride levels may not be connected to high levels of cholesterol in blood, nonetheless, lowering the triglyceride level does help to lower cholesterol.

Cholesterol is responsible for arteriosclerosis, heart attacks, and other illnesses. But it is essential for health. It is present in the skin and is converted to vitamin D in the presence of sunlight. It is a supplier of life-essential adrenalin and steroid hormones such as cortisone. It is necessary for the production of male and female sex hormones.

Two-thirds of the body's cholesterol is produced in the liver or intestines. A high cholesterol level in blood (>200 mg/100gm) is more likely to cause heart disease as compared to low or normal levels of cholesterol (<200 mg/100 gm). Therefore, the nutritional value of oils and fats must be taken into consideration for maintaining better health.

Vegetable Oils as a Source of Fat in Food:

Generally, fats and oils should not be directly consumed as food. But they are helpful as mediums of cooking for various vegetarian and non-vegetarian food preparations. Vegetable oil used in cooking improves the taste and flavor of foods. The oil also contains different vitamins and minerals and some essential fatty acids (EFA), which are required for maintaining better health.

Among the different vegetable oils, olive, groundnut, sesame, canola, cotton seed, and rice bran oils have more MUSF, hence, these oils are considered "good fats." However, these oils tend to increase the levels of both good cholesterol (HDL) and bad cholesterol (LDL) in blood. These oils also contain minerals like P, Ca, Mg and K along with vitamins like retinol, niacin, folic acid, tocopherol, etc. But it is low in vitamins B, C, and D. These oils are more stable for frequent frying and can be stored for periods of up to two years. Almond and peanut/groundnut oil also contain Vitamin E (tocopherol), which is important to the health of skin, hair, and brain.

Oils of sunflower, soybean, safflower, and corn, etc. contain more PUFA fatty acids like linoleic (EFA) and oleic. These oils are free from any toxic substance and are considered premium-quality food fats. They increase the level of HDL and decrease the level of LDL in blood. They also contain vitamin B complex, tocopherol, thymine, pantothenic acid, riboflavin, ascorbic acid, etc. However, these oils are not stable. They should not be used in frequent frying and cannot be stored for longer periods.

Oils of coconut, palm, and mustard contain more saturated fatty acids like linolenic, steric, etc. They are not considered good food fat, because these oils increase the level of LDL and decrease the level of HDL in blood. Mustard oil contains eurasic acid, which gives pungency to the oil but is harmful to health. These oils should be used in limited quantity.

Animal Products as Sources of Fat in Food:

Animal products like milk, meat, eggs, fish, etc. are sources of animal-produced food fat in human diets. Most of the animal-produced fats have more saturated fatty acids and can increase the level of LDL in blood. They are not considered good food fats with the exception of butter and cod-liver oil. This is because butter contains 10% butyric acid, which is easily digested and does not increase the level of LDL cholesterol. Similarly, cod-liver oil contains EFA, which lowers the level of LDL cholesterol.

(4) VITAMINS

Like carbohydrates, protein, and fats, vitamins are also important components of our daily foods for maintaining better health and strength. A deficiency of any vitamin can cause different diseases and disorders in the body. Vitamins are considered protective for better health. All of these vitamins: A, B Comp., C, D, E, and K are required for the proper functioning of various bio-physio processes within the body.

Most of these vitamins are available from our daily foods of cereals, legumes, fats, oils, spices, fresh fruits, dried fruits, vegetables, etc. So, the daily schedule of our foods should be formulated in such a way that we meet our requirements for vitamins.

Vitamin A (Retinol or Carotene):

Vitamin A is the most important vitamin for eye health. Deficiencies of this vitamin can cause night blindness or swelling of the eye.

Vitamin A from animal food sources is called retinol and Vitamin A from plant food sources is known as B-carotene. Retinol and B-carotene are converted into Vitamin A in the body. Vitamin A is synthesized in the intestinal flora of the body. Foods like carrot, green coriander, papaya, mango, peas, cantaloupe, oatmeal, golden rice, milk, meat, eggs, fish, etc. are rich in vitamin A content.

Vitamin B (Complex):

Vitamin B complex is made up of eight different types of vitamin B such as B-1 (Thiamine), B-2 (Riboflavin), B-3 (Niacin), B-5 (Pantothenic Acid), B-6 (Pyridoxine), B-7 (Biotin), B-9 (Folic acid), B-12 (Cabalamin). Each of the vitamins in the B-complex controls a specific bio-physio process within the body's systems.

A deficiency of vitamin B can cause loss of appetite, hair loss, and heart disease (B-5), brain and nerve disease, high blood pressure, coma, diabetes, heart and kidney diseases, birth defects (B-9), fertility disorders (B-12), etc.

Vitamin B is available from foods like legumes, cereals, nuts, soybeans, sunflowers, sesame, milk, eggs, meat, bananas, green vegetables, etc.

Vitamin C (Ascorbic Acid):

Vitamin C is important for the health of skin, gums, liver, kidney, etc. A deficiency of vitamin C can cause black and blue bruises on the skin, gum swelling, and loss of appetite.

It is present in large quantity in citrus fruits like lemon, grapefruit, or orange (89 mg), and in guava (228 mg), yellow bell pepper (180 mg), lychee (71 mg), kiwi (93 mg), mango, strawberry, tomato, grape, rose hip, spinach, cauliflower, etc.

Vitamin D (7-D Hydro cholesterol):

Vitamin D is important for the health of brain, nerve, and cardiac systems.

It is synthesized in large amounts in skin, kidney, bone, and liver when the body is exposed to early-morning sunlight. It is present in foods like soymilk, eggs, mushrooms, cod-liver oil, fish, etc.

Vitamin E (Tocopherol):

This is important for the health of skin, hair, heart, brain, nerves, etc. It is present in large quantity in nuts, papaya, mango, kiwi, canola oil, olive oil, avocado etc.

Vitamin K (Menadione):

This is important for blood clotting, bone strength, and regulation of metabolism, body temperature, etc. It is available in foods like carrot, kale, cabbage, winter squash (such as pumpkin and other mature squash), spinach, strawberry, etc.

(5) MINERALS

Minerals are very important components of our daily foods like carbohydrates, protein, fats, vitamins, and roughage. They are essential for the functioning of the various bio-physiological processes of our bodies. Therefore, a deficiency of any mineral can cause different diseases and disorders.

Minerals support the bio-physio processes in our body systems.

Two types of minerals are present in the body. The first type comprises macro minerals like calcium, chloride, magnesium, phosphorus, potassium, sodium, and sulfur, which are required in volume in our bodies. The others are trace minerals, such as iron, fluoride, and iodine, which are required in lower amounts in our bodies. The roles of these different minerals and their availability in our foods are given below.

Calcium:

Calcium is important for bone structure, teeth formation, cellular processes, muscle contraction, blood clotting, enzyme activation, regular heartbeat, impulse transmission, the nervous system, etc.

It is present in large amounts in foods like milk and milk products, broccoli, legumes, nuts or dried fruits, turnip, oysters, etc. Ca + P for strong and healthy bones and teeth as well as Ca + Mg for a healthier cardiovascular system.

Chloride:

It is an essential mineral element for primary ionization, maintenance of pH balance, and enzyme activation, and it is a component of gastric hydrochloric acid. Deficiency can cause discoloration of hair and teeth. It is available in large amounts in table salt, seafood, milk, meat, eggs, etc.

Magnesium:

It is a component of bones and teeth and helps in nerve-impulse transmission and protein synthesis, supporting the cardiovascular system. It is available in large amounts in nuts, legumes, cereals, soybeans, peas, carrots, brown rice, seafoods, etc.

Phosphorus:

It is a structural component of bone and teeth. It is also an important component of membrane, phospholipids, nucleic acid, nucleotides, ATP, ADP, phosphatic transfer, and pH regulation. Deficiency causes rickets and pyorrhea.

It is available in large amounts from foods like nuts, legumes, cereals, milk and milk products, meat, fish, eggs, etc.

Potassium:

It helps in the maintenance of balance in water, electrolytes, and pH, and it also helps in cell membrane transmission. It is present in large amounts in foods like avocado, banana, orange, peas, potato, tomato, beans, nuts, wheat, soybean, eggs, dairy products, etc.

Sodium:

It helps in water, electrolyte, and pH regulation; nerve transmission; muscle construction; and prevents sun stroke, heat prostration, and blood pressure problems. It is available in table salt, and foods like seafood, garlic, meat, dairy products, vegetables, etc.

Sulfur:

It is essential for healthy hair, skin, and nails; it helps in dietary function; and it is also required to build amino acids. Sulfur is one of the elements required to produce enzymes like thymine and biotin.

Ferric:

It is important for the synthesis of hemoglobin in blood cells and the liver. A deficiency can cause pale skin and pale lips. It carries oxygen to different parts of the body. It is available in large amounts in cabbage, cauliflower, eggs, papaya, black plum, beans, milk, etc.

Iodine:

A deficiency of iodine can cause hypothyroid, dry skin, thin hair, hair loss, muscle weakness, goiter, birth defects, miscarriage, premature birth, weight gain, feeling cold, and irregular periods. Iodine is available in corn, strawberries, bananas, green beans, eggs, milk, meat, salt, and seafood.

Fluoride:

Fluoride is important for the health of teeth. It is available from tea, fish, water, strawberries, etc.

Manganese:

Manganese is an essential element, which helps in impulse transmission and protein synthesis. It improves memory, protects against osteoporosis, and eliminates fatigue.

Selenium:

Selenium and Vitamin E are synergistic; they are required for males, because they are lost in semen.

Zinc:

Zinc helps in insulin formation, protein synthesis, construction of muscles, and production of reproductive cells. It can help to prevent some prostate problems and mental disorders. It works best with Vitamin A and minerals Ca and P.

Vitamins absorb more efficiently in the presence of different minerals as shown below:

Vitamins	Minerals
Vitamin A	Ca, Mg, P, S, Z
Vitamin B	Cu, Cob, Fe, Mn, K, Na
Vitamin C	Ca, Cob, Cu, Fe, Na
Vitamin D	Ca, Cu, Mg, Se, Na
Vitamin E	Ca, Fe, Mn, P, K, Sa, Na, Zn

Therefore, food combinations should be arranged in such a way that vitamins and minerals are consumed together.

Vegetables and Fruits as Sources of Vitamins and Minerals in Food:

Vegetables and fruits are the principle source of vitamins and minerals in our food. Therefore, about 200 grams of vegetables and 250 grams of fruits are required per day in our daily diets, to provide enough vitamins and minerals to maintain our health and the strength of our bodies.

Often, vegetables like cabbage, cauliflower, broccoli, spinach, tomato, carrot, beet, radish, onion, peppers, lettuce, cucumbers, etc. are consumed as green salad. Vegetables like potato, eggplant, gourds, okra, etc. are consumed as cooked vegetables. Coriander leaves, ginger, turmeric, garlic, chilies, etc. are consumed as spices in small quantity. Green legumes like peas, pigeon peas, beans, lentils, black-eyed peas, etc. are consumed as whole grains. Green legumes contain more vitamins and minerals. Fresh vegetables brought from market or field should be washed thoroughly and stored in the refrigerator. Such fresh-picked vegetables retain more vitamins and minerals.

As opposed to Teflon or metals like aluminum, the cooking of vegetables in stainless steel or glass or enamel cookware helps in retaining more vitamins and minerals. The shorter the cooking time and the less water used in cooking, the lower the loss of vitamins and minerals. Using a sharp knife and not cutting vegetables until just before you use them also helps prevent the loss of vitamins and minerals.

Commercially produced fruit juice often contains added water and sugar. Fresh fruits are more nutritious and should be prepared at home.

Fruits like orange, lemon, grapefruits, etc. can be consumed as fresh juice or as cut pieces. They contain Vitamin C and minerals like Ca, P, K, Mg, Fe, etc. Fruits like orange, mango, guava, pomegranate, papaya, banana, watermelon, muskmelon, pineapple, etc. can also be juiced or consumed in cut pieces. They contain Vitamin A, B, C, and minerals like Ca, P, K, Fe, Mg, S, etc.

Small fruits like blueberry, blackberry, raspberry, grapes, kiwi, strawberry, black plum, sapota, etc. can also be consumed as juice or whole fruits. They contain Vitamin C and minerals like Ca, P, K, Fe, Mg, etc.

Nutritional Components in Fruits

Nutritional components	Fruits					
	Mango	Papaya	Straw-berry	Water-melon	Fig	Coconut
Water (%)	81.0	80.8	87.8	92.0	88.1	93.8
Carbohydrate (%)	17.0	7.2	9.8	3.3	0.6	4.4
Protein (%)	0.6	0.6	0.7	0.2	1.3	-
Fat (%)	0.4	0.1	0.2	0.2	0.2	0.1
Calories	74	32	44	30	37	-
Mineral (mg/100 gm)						
Potassium	20.0	19.0	-	16.0	0.8	-
Calcium	14.0	17.0	30.0	7.0	8.0	-
Phosphorus	16.0	13.0	30.0	12.0	3.0	-
Ferric	1.3	0.5	1.8	7.9	1.0	-
Sodium	26.0	6.0	-	-	-	0.1
Vitamins (mg/100 gm)						
Vitamin A (carotene)	274.0	666.0	18.0	-	100.0	-
Vitamin B1 (Thymine)	0.9	0.4	0.3	-	0.06	-
Vitamin B2 (Riboflavin)	0.9	0.2	0.2	-	0.01	10.0
Vitamin B3 (Niacin)	16.0	0.2	2.0	-	0.60	100.0
Vitamin C	21.0	59.0	52.0	-	5.0	2.0

(6) ROUGHAGE (FIBER):

Like carbohydrates, protein, fat, mineral, and vitamins, roughage is also one of the important nutritional components of food. Roughage is also called fiber. About 30-35 grams of fiber are required for adults per day. Most of the fiber is available from plant food. Fiber does not provide any nutrients but can help to prevent diseases or infection. Therefore, for healthy, longer lives, people should eat some coarse foods that contain indigestible fiber. All fiber is not the same, but various types perform the different functions shown below.

Cellulose and hemicellulose absorb water and help in the smooth functioning of the large intestine. As a result, waste can move through the colown more rapidly. Thus, they can prevent constipation, and this lowers cholesterol levels and prevents other diseases. The fiber found in cereal brans like wheat and corn is insoluble while soluble fiber is found in rice, oat, and barley and is found in carrots, apples, broccoli, peas, cabbage, cucumber, etc.

Gum and pectin also influence water absorption in the stomach and small intestine where they reduce fat and sugar absorption. As a result, cholesterol level is reduced, and less insulin is needed. This kind of fiber is found in foods like oatmeal, carrots, cabbage, cauliflower, apples, citrus fruits, peas, beans, potatoes, etc.

Another fiber, **lignin,** is found in vegetables like eggplant, green beans, radish, etc., and it reduces the digestibility of other fiber also. As a result, cholesterol level goes down.

However, too much fiber intake causes gas, vomiting, and diarrhea and reduces the absorption of certain minerals like calcium, phosphorus, magnesium, iron, zinc, etc.

(7) WATER

Water is also considered one of the nutritional components of food. (Approximately fifty to eighty percent of our body weight is water. It is the basic solvent for digestion of all foods. It is also essential for the moving of waste in all the systems of the body. It is advisable to drink about three to four liters of water daily for better health. Hot water dissolves more lead than cold water does. Therefore, one should avoid drinking hot water. Water mixed with more than the required amount of chloride or contaminated with pesticide should not be used even for shower purposes. Everyday drinking water, which is available from home water-filtering systems, reverse-osmosis systems (RO), or distillers has some drawbacks. If water has not been pre-processed for disinfection (such as through chlorination), then this water should be boiled at least for twenty minutes to remove the pathogens and harmful chemicals. Then this water should be cooled and safely stored, before being used for drinking purposes.

II. FOOD PREPARATIONS FOR VARIOUS NUTRITIONAL COMPONENTS

Carbohydrates:

In order to meet the personal requirement of 150 to 200 grams of carbohydrates per day in our daily food, about 200 to 250 grams of any grain cereal in the form of flour, whole grain, or brans should be used in food preparation in any regional diet. These preparations can be used by vegetarians and non-vegetarians alike.

Grain Cereals	Form or Sub-product	Final food preparations for eating
Wheat	Flour	Bread, Pizza, Pasta, Noodles, Cake, Biscuits, Cookies, etc.
Rice	Flour	Various breads, rice dishes, wraps etc.
	Whole grain	Steam cooked, or boiled rice eaten with legumes or vegetables, or meat or fish, etc.
Maize	Flour	Baked breads, steam cooked, etc.
	Whole grain	Popcorn or Bran, etc.
	Immature seeds	Steam cooked, sweet corn as whole grain or soup, etc.
Millet Sorghum	Flour	Breads or steam cooked, etc.
	Whole grain	Roasted or steam cooked, etc.

Protein:

To meet the requirement of 50 grams of protein per day in our daily diet, 25 grams of protein can be contributed by cereal food and the remaining 25 grams of protein should be obtained from the consumption of 100 grams of any grain legumes. Grain legumes can be in the form of flour, whole or split grains, or immature seeds, etc. They are used for a variety of food preparations as shown below:

Grain Legumes	Form or Sub-product	Final food preparations for eating
Soybean	Flour	It is blended with wheat flour for making multi-grain bread, pizza, etc.
	Whole grain	Steam cooked and eaten after mixing with vegetables and spices, etc.
Peas	Whole grain	Steam cooked with vegetables and spices. than eaten with breads, etc.
Pigeon pea	Split grain	Steam cooked with salt and spices, till they become soft and semi liquid. Then eaten with rice, bread, etc.
	Immature seeds	Use as vegetable or mixed vegetables, etc.
Black-eyed peas	Matured grain	Steam cooked with salt and spices and eaten with rice, bread, etc.
	Immature grains and pods	Use as green vegetables or mixed vegetables, etc.
Mung beans or Black beans	Whole grain or split grain (dal)	Steam cooked with salt and spices then eaten with rice, bread, etc.
Chickpea	Flour	Fried food preparations, etc.
	Whole grain	Steam cooked or roasted with salt and spices, etc.

Oils and Fats:

Generally, about 50 grams of oil and fats are required per day in our diets. Oils or fats are used as a cooking medium in making various food preparations from cereals to legumes or vegetables according to the food habits of people in different countries. The qualities of different food fats are given below:

Oils / Fats	Food fats quality	Properties
Ground nut, Sesame, Cotton-seed, Rice bran, Canola	Good	Oils contain equal amounts of SFA, MUFA, and PUFA. Therefore, they do not increase the level of LDL choles-terol in blood. Suitable for frequent frying and long periods of storage.
Sunflower, Saf-flower, Soybean, Niger seed, Corn	Premium and good	Oils contain more USFA like olive and Linoleic (EFA), which increase the level of HDL cholesterol in the blood. Good for cooking but not for frequent frying. These oils are more oxidative and hence should not be stored for long periods.
Mustard, Coconut, Palm	Not good food fat	Oils contain more SFA, which increases the level of LDL cholesterol in blood
Animal fat such as Butter, Ghee	Good food fat	These contain more SFA but also contain 10% butyric acid, which helps to regulate the level of LDL in the blood.
Animal fat, Meat, Egg	Not good food fat	These contain more SFA, which increases the level of LDL in the blood.

Note: SFA (Saturated Fatty Acid), MUFA (Monounsaturated Fatty Acid), PUFA (Poly Unsaturated Fatty Acid), EFA (Essential Fatty Acid)

Vitamins and Minerals:

In order to obtain the required quantity of vitamins and minerals for maintaining proper health and strength, about

200 grams of vegetables and 250 grams of fruits are required in our daily diets. Vegetables can be consumed in the form of salad or can be steam cooked or ground like whole grains, etc. Fruits can be consumed in the form of juice, cut pieces, whole fruit, or jam and jelly.

Name of vegetable / fruits	Form of consumption	Availability	
		Vita-mins	Minerals
Cabbage, Cauliflower, Carrot, Beet, Radish, Broccoli, Tomato, Onion, Beet, Peppers, Lettuce, Spinach	Salad	A, B, C, K	Ca, P, K, Fe, Mg
Eggplant, Potato, Gourds, Okra, Sweet Potato	Cooked vegetables	A, B, C	Ca, P, K, Fe, Mg
Ginger, Turmeric, Garlic, Onion, Coriander	Ground up or small pieces	A, B, C	Ca, P, K, S, Fe, Mg
Green legumes like Peas, Black-eyed Peas, Pigeon Peas, Lentils, Beans, Chickpeas	Whole grain	A, B, C	Ca, P, K, S, Fe, Mg
Cluster Beans, Black-eyed Peas, Beans, Lentils	Green pods	A, K	Ca, P, K, S, Fe, Mg
Orange, Lemon, Grape, Grapefruit	Juice	A, C	Ca, P, K, Fe, Mg, S
Apple, Guava, Pomegranate, Pineapple, Papaya, Pears, Mango, Watermelon, Muskmelon, Avocado, Sapota	Cut pieces or juice	A, B, C	Ca, P, K, Fe, Mg
Strawberry, Blueberry, Raspberry, Kiwi, Grape, Blackplum, Cherry	Whole fruit	A, B, C	Ca, P, K, Fe, Mg

III. MEDICINAL HERBAL FOODS

SPICES AND CONDIMENTS are food materials, which are mixed in small quantities with vegetarian and non-vegetarian food preparations at the time of cooking to improve and enhance taste, flavors, digestibility, and palatability. Spices are generally ground into small pieces or powder form. Spices like cardamom, cloves, cinnamon, black pepper, cumin, coriander, caraway, celery seed, fennel, fenugreek, etc. contain specific types of oil, which create aroma. Chilies, ginger, turmeric, etc. are also used as spices. All these spices contain nutrients like carbohydrates, protein, fats, vitamins, minerals, roughage, and specific medicinal substances in various amounts.

The dry, powder form of the seeds of plants like cumin, caraway, dill, coriander, fennel, black pepper, fenugreek, sesame, etc. is used in spice. All these spices have different tastes, aromas, and specific medicinal properties. They can be used for taking care of indigestion, gastritis, acidity, constipation, bad breath, and vomiting.

Crops like ginger, turmeric, garlic, onion, etc. are use as spices in the form of powdered, matured, and dried stems, as well as small pieces of immature and green stems. All these

31

spices have different tastes, aromas, and specific medicinal properties. They can used to take care of the common cold, cough, flu, gastritis, heart disease, mental depression, etc.

Spice crops like cardamom, cloves, nutmeg, etc. are used as spices in the form of whole dried fruit or the powder of dried fruits. All these spices have different tastes, aromas, and specific medicinal properties. They can be used in the care of tooth pain, gum swelling, bad breath, indigestion, headaches, appetite loss, infertility, vomiting, etc.

IV. NUTS / DRIED FRUIT FOODS

NUTS AND DRIED FRUIT are the most important foods among all the plant-based or animal-based foods, because they are more nutritious, digestible, and healthy foods. Most nuts like cashew, almond, walnut, or pistachio, or dried fruit like raisins, apricots, dates, figs, berries, etc. are consumed whole or in cut pieces. They can also be consumed as powder or small pieces by mixing with milk products, sweets, and other food preparations. Nuts and dried fruits contain good quality nutrients like carbohydrates, protein, fats, vitamins, minerals, and other medicinal substances. Oils from almond, cashew, pistachio, walnut, etc. provide good quality fat (MUFA), which increases HDL in blood cholesterol. Most nuts and dried fruits can act as brain tonics because they contain good quality fat and protein along with sufficient quantities of vitamins and minerals. They can also detoxify blood and body. Generally, 10 grams of nuts or dried fruits should be consumed per day for better health and strength.

Food Components of Dried Fruits and Nuts

Nutritional Components	Dried Fruits and Nuts				
	Cashew	Almond	Pistachio	Raisin	Figs
Carbohydrate (%)	28.3	10.5	26.8	74.6	70.6
Protein (%)	21.2	20.8	26.4	1.8	1.8
Fat (%)	51.0	58.9	46.5	0.3	1.3
Calories	646	655	568	308	325

Nuts and dried fruits have high nutritive value, because most of them are rich in good-quality food fat, protein, and carbohydrates along with important vitamins and minerals. Therefore, they should be eaten in appropriate quantities.

Nuts like walnut, peanut, cashew, pistachio, etc. are consumed either raw or roasted in the form of dried whole kernels or as the powder of dried kernels. The oil of most of these nuts has high amounts of mono-unsaturated fatty acid, which increases HDL and reduces cholesterol level in blood.

Dried fruits like raisins, dates, and figs are rich in high-quality carbohydrates, vitamins, and minerals. They help to maintain the hemoglobin in blood.

V. FOODS FOR STAYING YOUNG

PEOPLE OFTEN WANT TO LOOK YOUNGER than their actual age. Aging is a natural process caused by the continuous degeneration of body cells, which have the life span of less than two years. Every cell reproduces itself before it dies, but the body becomes older as time passes and we age.

Anti-aging Nutrients for Looking Younger:

Research conducted on the effects of nucleic acid therapy on aging has indicated that nucleic acid treatment rejuvenates the deteriorated cells by direct nourishment, slowing down or ceasing the formation of new cells. As a result, a body can look five to ten years younger than its actual age. Moreover, the enzyme superoxide dismutase (SOD), taken with a natural diet, slows down the aging process by restricting the formation of free radicals, which are responsible for speeding up the aging process by destroying healthy cells.

However, when age is advanced, the body produces less superoxide dismutase (SOD). Superoxide dismutase (SOD) also becomes less active in the absence of essential nutrients like Zn, Cu, and Mn. So, foods that are rich in nucleic acid and Zn, like wheat, corn, bran, spinach, asparagus, mushroom, fish, chicken, oatmeal, onion, etc. should be eaten regularly.

Synthesized from three amino acids like L-cysteine, L-glutamine acid, and glycine, which act as antioxidants and deactivate free radicals, tripeptide glutathione is responsible for slowing down the process of aging. Likewise, sulfur amino acid cystine is also important as an anti-aging nutrient. All these nutrients are available from protein-rich foods like legumes, soybeans, dairy products, eggs, meat, nuts, fish, etc.

Energetic Nutrients for Better Sex:

It has been found that male potency and fertility increase due to nutrients like vitamin-E and minerals like Zn. Both these nutrients are helpful in raising energy levels along promoting a stronger sex drive. Amino acids like arginine, lysine, and tyrosine also help in increasing fertility and sex drive. Eaten either raw or lightly cooked, foods like wheat germ, wheat bran, whole grains, barley, brown rice, sunflower seeds, onion, oyster, and shellfish, along with other energizing foods rich in vitamin-B and amino acids, are found to be helpful as well. Garlic provides sulfur compounds to the body. Sulfur improves the protection of skin and enhances its growth. It is also critical for skin elasticity. In this way, sulfur improves appearance. Eating dates with ghee increases sex drive in men. Mixing Indian gooseberry with other herbal medicinal nutrients is energy enhancing and improves sex drive in both men and women.

VI. FOODS FOR BETTER APPEARANCE

BEAUTY IN WOMEN or a handsome appearance in men is a gift of nature. But it can be manipulated to some extent with the use of different chemical and herbal beauty products. For better health and an improved appearance, people take external and internal care of their skin, hair, nails, hands, and feet for better health. Among the products used are herbal oils, ointments, creams, lotions, shampoos, conditioners, face wash, etc., which are used externally. But natural foods are also very effective in improving outward appearance.

For Healthy and Glowing Skin:

Healthy and glowing skin improves the appearance of both men and women. Manufacturers of beauty products make many claims as to their effectiveness, and so, many people take care of their skin externally with chemical and herbal beauty products. Some people though suffer from various skin diseases like acne; black heads; red spots; white heads; corns; calluses; dermatitis; eczema; dry, rough, scaly skin; etc. Healthy, glowing skin cannot be created and maintained through external means only; it requires internal nourishment with nutrients like Vitamin E, A, B2, B3, B6, and B7 as well as chelated minerals like, Cu, Zn, I, Fe, S, K, etc., which are essential. For obtaining all these nutrients, foods like protein drinks, herbal teas, non-fat milk, yeast, banana, strawberry, orange, papaya, carrot, fish, eggs, and omega-3 sources like flax seed, canola oil, soybean oil, walnut, and sunflower seeds must be eaten regularly.

For Strong and Shiny Hair:

For an attractive look, healthy, shiny, strong hair is the first preference of both men and women. That's why people use so many brands of hair oil, lotions, creams, shampoos, conditioners, hair coloring, etc. for the external treatment of their hair. Meanwhile they may be suffering from problems like hair loss; graying; dull, dry, or brittle hair; dandruff; etc. Thus, it is essential to treat hair internally with specific nutrients like Vitamin B5, B6, B7, B9, B12, unsaturated fatty acids like linoleic, linolenic, and arachidonic and minerals like sulfur, calcium, iodine, and chlorine, etc. To obtain these nutrients, natural foods like yeast, almonds, peanuts, walnuts, dairy products, iodized salt, green vegetables, citrus fruits, broccoli, cabbage, tomatoes, meats, eggs, fish, etc. should be eaten regularly.

Hair should be regularly washed with protein-rich shampoo and scalps massaged with Vitamin E-rich oil from almond, jojoba, etc.

For Healthy Hands, Feet, and Nails:

Hands and feet are the most active parts of our bodies and throughout life regularly work in all the extremes of weather. People use various types of gloves and shoes as well as different oils, ointments, creams, lotion, hand-soaps, etc. for external protection. But hands and feet may suffer from problems like splitting nails, brittle nails, white strips and spots on nails, skin peeling on hands, and rough and hard skin like corns, etc. Internal care should be provided by taking in specific nutrients like vitamin E, C, B6, and B9 as well as minerals like Zn, I, Silica, etc. All these nutrients are available from foods like wheat germ, wheat bran, green vegetables, grains, sunflower seeds, yeast, eggs, nuts, etc.

Beside this, hands, feet, and nails can be kept smooth and soft with regular massage using herbal oils, ointments, creams, or lotions.

VII. FOOD FOR FIT, HEALTHY BODIES

PEOPLE SOMETIMES SUFFER from different diseases and disorders throughout their lives. Some are affected in childhood, some in youth, and some in old age. Nutrient deficiency may be a cause of some of these diseases and disorders. That's why it is advised to nutritionally balance one's diet from childhood to old age to enjoy a happy and healthy life. Better nutrition acts as a preventive measure against many diseases and disorders.

Every individual wants to maintain a fit body throughout life. A fit body is the proper harmony between height and weight, which is controlled by hormones secreted by the thyroid gland. To maintain proper functioning of the thyroid gland, enough iodine and manganese must be consumed. Natural foods like salt, seafood, fish liver oil, corn, strawberries, green beans, bananas, milk, meat, eggs, fish, etc. should be eaten regularly.

A fit body should have healthy skin, hair, and nails maintained with internal and external care. Nutrients like Vitamin E, C, B5 and B9, protein drinks for amino acids, and minerals like Ca, Cu, Fe, K, Cl and Zn are essential to obtain these nutrients. Foods like yeast, milk, almonds, peanuts, walnuts, iodized salt, green vegetables, citrus fruits, bananas, broccoli, cabbage, tomatoes, soybean oil, canola oil, etc., should be eaten regularly. Lotion, ointment, shampoo, soap, cream, etc. made of aloe vera or jojoba and almond oils, etc. can be used externally.

Strong and healthy teeth and bones are also important in a fit and healthy body. Therefore, nutrients like Vitamin A and D as well as minerals like Ca, P, Mg, Mn, chlorine, iodine, and fluoride must be taken in regularly. All these nutrients are available in foods like milk and milk products, fish, liver oil, grain legumes, nuts, eggs, meat, green vegetables, mushrooms, carrots, etc. which should be consumed regularly.

A healthy nose, eyes, and ears, make our senses sharp and are indicators of a fit and healthy body. Nutrients like Vitamin A, B1, C, K, etc. and minerals like Zn, Mn, K, etc. are required for the proper functioning of our eyes, ears, and nose. Foods like cereals, legumes, nuts, milk and milk products, fish, eggs, green vegetables, carrot, citrus fruits, etc. should be eaten regularly.

A healthy heart and brain give super performance to a fit body. High levels of cholesterol and blood pressure should be avoided, otherwise they can cause heart disease. Nutrients like Vitamin A, C, B5, B7, B6, B12, chlorine, etc. as well as minerals like Ca, S, Mg, K, Zn, etc., along with amino acids like glutamine and glutamine acid, methionine, tyrosine, etc. are essential. Foods like olive oil, canola oil, garlic, onion, yeast, cod-liver oil, nuts, brans, avocados, and citrus fruits must be eaten regularly. Meanwhile, saturated fat and excessive amounts of salt and sugar should be avoided.

The reproductive organs, fertility, and sex hormones play an important role in maintaining a healthy body. Nutrients like Vitamin B1, B2, B9, B12, E, etc. and minerals like selenium, Zn etc. are essential. So, foods like seafood, fish, onions, eggs, tomatoes, broccoli, nuts, and carrots, must be eaten regularly.

Digestive-system problems like indigestion, gastritis, acidity, appetite loss, stomach fatigue, etc. can decrease the efficiency of the body systems. Nutrients like Vitamin A, B1, B2, B5, B9, etc., as well as multiple minerals are essential; they can be obtained from foods like cereals, nuts, legumes, green leafy vegetables, citrus fruits, yeast, eggs, fish, bananas, raisins, cauliflower, chilies, spinach, etc.

Taking in the above health factors, we have prepared a food schedule for a one-week period, as shown below. In this schedule the nutritional requirements are the same for all the different countries of the world, however, food preparations may be different.

Weekly food schedule for a fit and healthy body:

Nutri-ent	Carbohydrate (200 gm)	Protein (50 gm)	Fat (50 gm)	Vitamins / Minerals (as required)	
Foods Days	Grain cereals (250 gm) / Wheat / Rice / Maize / Millet	Grain legumes (100 gm) / Milk (500 ml), Meat / eggs/ fish (50 gm)	Oils / Butter / Ghee (50 gm)	Vege-tables (200 gm)	Fruits (250 gm)
Monday	Bread / Pizza / Burger / Boiled Rice / Noodle / Maize bran	Pigeon peas, Mung beans (WG), oats, cheese, meat, eggs, fish, milk	MUFA/ PUFA/ butter, Ghee	Cauli-flower, green peas, spinach, potato, garlic, salad, CCCBOT*	Apple, orange, papaya, black-berry, avocado

Tuesday	- same as above -	Pigeon peas, Chickpea (WG), yogurt, cheese, meat, eggs, fish, milk	-same as above-	Broccoli, garlic, green pigeon pea, calabash, fenu-greek leaves, sweet potato, salad, CCCBOT	Guava, canta-loupe, straw-berry, rasp-berry, lemon
Wed-nesday	- same as above -	Chickpeas, Dried peas (WG) yogurt, cheese, meat, eggs, fish, milk	-same as above-	Eggplant, garlic, green beans, bitter gourds, spinach, potato, salad, CCCBOT	Apple, grape-fruit, papaya, water-melon, grape
Thurs-day	- same as above -	Lentils, Green beans (WG), yogurt, cheese, meat, eggs, fish, milk	-same as above-	Okra, garlic, green peas, butter, sweet potato, salad, CCCBOT	Pine-apple, pom-egranate, cherry, mango, lemon
Friday	- same as above -	Pigeon peas, red kidney beans (WG), yogurt, cheese, meat, eggs, fish, milk	-same as above-	Cauli-flower, green leaf spinach, ridge gourd, potato, garlic, salad, CCCBOT	Apple, kiwi, straw-berry, banana, lemon

Satur-day	- same as above -	Soybeans, red kidney beans (WG), yogurt, cheese, meat, eggs, fish, milk	-same as above-	Broccoli, green pigeon peas, celery, salad, CCCBOT	Banana, grape, blue-berry, lemon
Sunday	- same as above -	Mung beans, moth bean or dew bean (WG), yogurt, cheese, milk	-same as above-	Eggplant, garlic, green fenu-greek, leaves, salad, CCCBOT	Orange, papaya, pearl, cheese, lemon

*WG (Whole grain), CCC (carrot, cabbage, cucumber), O (Onion), R (Radish), T (Tomato), B (Beet)

VIII. HERBAL REMEDIES

Basil (*Ocimum sanctum Linn.*):
Basil is an important medicinal plant and its leaves are used for the treatment of many external and internal diseases and disorders. A syrup prepared from its leaves is used for controlling the flu and the common cold. A poultice made of its leaves is used for alleviating white spots in the skin, blood impurities, pimples, and the poison generated by bee stings.

Aloe Vera (*Aloe barbadensis Mill.*):
This is a fleshy plant used for external and internal treatment of many diseases and disorders of the body. In addition to being found in shampoo and conditioners, Aloe Vera products like gels, oils, ointments, creams, lotions, etc. are used in the treatment of problems like pimples, burns, insect stings, blistering, peeling, corns, calluses, hemorrhoids, etc.

Alfalfa (*Medicago sativa*):
This is a legumin plant and its leaves contain eight essential enzymes; vitamins like A, B6, D, E, K, etc.; and minerals like Ca, Cu, P, etc. It protects against hemorrhaging and it helps in blood clotting. It supports strong bones and teeth in growing children. It is also used in the treatment of stomach pain, gas pain, poor appetite, ulcers, etc. It is a good laxative and diuretic.

Dill (*Anethum graveloens*):

The seed of this plant is useful for different remedies. It is a natural diuretic and gastric stimulant. It also improves appetite and digestion. It is used to relieve flatulence.

Garlic (*Allium sativum*):

Garlic is used as a spice for increasing taste and flavor in vegetarian and non-vegetarian food preparations in almost all the countries of the world. However, it is also a valuable herbal medicinal food. It contains good amounts of protein, vitamin B and C, and minerals like calcium, phosphorus, and potassium. It reduces blood pressure and lowers cholesterol and blood sugar. It also alleviates grippe, sore throat, etc. Garlic provides sulfur compounds to the body. Sulfur improves the protection and growth of skin. It is also critical for skin elasticity, which preserves beauty. The eating of dates with ghee increases sex drive in men. Mixing Indian gooseberry with other herbal medicinal nutrients is energy enhancing and improves sex drive in both men and women.

Kelp:

Kelp is a seaweed and contains more vitamins and minerals than many other foods. Kelp has a lot of iodine in it and so it aids the thyroid gland by increasing the weight of thin people and reducing the weight of the obese. It can also be used in the treatment of poor digestion, flatulence, constipation, etc.

Algae:

Blue-green algae (spirulina) and emerald algae (chlorella) belong to the plant kingdom. They are easily assimilated complete protein. They contain natural chlorophyll and are rich in vitamin A, B, C, and E as well as minerals like Ca, K, Mg and Zn, which help in reducing weight, healing wounds, and decreasing the pain of arthritis.

Ajani (*Trachyspermum ammi*):

The seeds of this plant are used for various remedies. The oil or powder of the seeds is used to induce vomiting, and to treat the common cold, coughs, loss of appetite, etc.

Hing (*Fetula assafoctida*):

The gum secreted by the asafetida plant is processed and used for various remedies. The powder prepared from the dried gum is used as a spice in food preparation as well as in the preparation of various herbal medicines. It helps in the curing of gastritis, acidity, indigestion, etc.

Nutmeg (*Myristica fragrans*):

The dried fruit of this tree is used for different remedies. Nutmeg powder is used for treating pimples, the common cold, indigestion, headaches, sleeplessness, diarrhea, etc.

Saffron (*Corcus sativus*):

The long, thin pollen tube of the saffron flower (saffron thread) has a vivid color and a lotus-like smell. The threads are dissolved either in milk or water and added to various food preparations and herbal medicines. Saffron helps in alleviating thought disorders, skin diseases, cold and cough, etc.

Indian Gooseberry (*Emblica officinalis Gaertu*):

The ripened fruits of this tree contain high amounts of vitamin C, minerals, and iron. They are used for various food preparations like juice, jam, jelly, pickles, etc. Indian gooseberry is a good remedy for increasing energy and immunity.

Vinea Rosea (*Catharanthus roseas*):

This is a beautiful, small, and profusely flowering plant. The plant can have white, purple, pink, or red flowers. It grows in all the seasons of the year. Its dried leaves and roots are used for the treatment of different diseases including cancer.

Bhangro (*Edipta postrata*):

This is a small plant, which bears white flowers and black seeds. The green plant is more useful as compared to dried. It is used for treating hair, skin, the liver, the eyes, and dental diseases.

Indian Senna (*Cassia Angustifolia vahl*):

The plant contains sennosides, which are used in remedies for certain diseases. Dry leaves can be used in preparation of suru (powder), tablets, or capsules for stomach diseases and cough.

Jethimadh (*Glycyrrhiza glabra*):

The root of this plant is used for various remedies like the alleviating of cough, mouth sores, and bronchitis, and for improving fertility in males.

Winter Cherry (*Withania somnitera*):

The powder made from the roots of this plant is used for different remedies. It stimulates physical and mental energy and is known as the "Indian ginseng." It also helps increase milk production in lactating mothers and is used to treat various skin diseases.

Mitho Limdo (*Murraya koengii*):
The green as well as the dried leaves of this shrub are used for various remedies. It is used to treat certain skin diseases. It also lends good taste and flavor to various food preparations, and it improves digestion.

Jojoba (*Jetropha Curcab*):
The oil extracted from the seeds of the jojoba plant is used in the preparation of ointments, creams, lotions, shampoos, etc., which are used in remedies for skin and hair conditions.

Kuvadio (*Cassia tora*):
The powdered form of the dried roots or a syrup made from the roots is used for clearing up some skin diseases.

Aradusi (*Adhatoda Vasica*):
This is an evergreen shrub and the leaves are used for various remedies. The juice or a paste prepared from fresh leaves is used for treating colds, coughs, flu, bronchitis, T.B., etc.

Creat (*Andrgraphis paniculata Burmf*):
This is an important herbal plant used for treating cold, cough, fever, skin diseases, indigestion, diabetes, etc.

IX. FOODS / NUTRIENTS THAT CAN BE SUBSTITUTED FOR DRUGS

Drugs	Food / Nutrients
Antacids	Papaya, Dill, Ajwain, Mint, Coriander, Pineapple, Citrus Medicago Glycine, Multiple Digestive enzymes
Anticoagulant	Almond, Peanut, Walnut, Wheat Germ, Avocado, Apple, Vitamin E, Pectin
Antibiotic	Turmeric, Garlic, Cabbage Vitamin A, B, C, B9, C
Antidepressants	Pistachio, Apple, Papaya, Grape, Cassia Tora, Gotu Kola Vitamin B1, B3, B6, B11, Choline, Tyrosine, Tryptophan, L-phenylamine
Antidiarrhoeic	Yogurt, Pomegranate Pulp, Vitamin B3, Lactobacillus Acidophilus
Diuretic	Watermelon, Alfalfa, Dill, Onion, Yeast, Parsley, Black Plum, Gotu Kola, Sapodilla, Asparagus, Indian Gooseberry, Strawberry Vitamin B6, E
Laxative	Alfalfa, Brans, Nutmeg, Castor Oil Vitamin B1, B2, B6, B12, Calcium

Anticancer	Carrot, Pumpkin, Sweet Potato, Papaya, Cantaloupe, Cruciferous Vegetables Vitamin C, Selenium
Antidandruff	Legumes, Cereals, Sunflower Seeds, Peanuts, Walnuts, Milk, Meat, Eggs, Fish, Broccoli, Onions, Tomatoes, Gotu Kola, Eclipta Alba Vitamin B6, B12, Selenium
Antigastritis	Garlic, Dill, Caraway, Legumes, Nuts, Milk, Yeast, Sapodilla, Citrus Fruits, Tomato, Kelp, Cardamom Vitamin B1, B2, B6, B9, Glycine
Antioxidant	Spinach, Blackberry, Cauliflower, Cabbage, Green Chili, Walnut, Broccoli Vitamin A (carotine), C, E, Selenium, L-glutathione
Antidiabetic	Black Plum, Cluster Bean, Wheat, Soybean, Fenugreek, Creat, Bitter Gourd, B15
Antiosteoporosis	Boron with Ca, Mg and Vitamin D, Milk, Soybean, Peanut, Walnut, Banana, Kola, Broccoli
Anti- inflammatory	Spinach, Strawberry, Legumes, Cereals, Nuts, Yeast, Meat, Fish, Egg Vitamin B2, B6, B7, B3
Antiaging	Wheat Germ, Brans, Spinach, Asparagus, mushroom, Fish, Oatmeal, Onion, Seafood, Milk, Fruit, or Vegetable Juice Collagen, Nucleic acid, Superoxide Dismutase, Vitamin E.

X. SPECIFIC HEALTH FOODS

FOODS LIKE CABBAGE, cauliflower, broccoli, radish, squash, kale, celery, etc. of the cruciferous family; nutrients like Vitamin E; and minerals such as Selenium are potent and good inhibitors of cancer-producing carcinogens.

Foods like olive oil and carrot are effective against heart diseases.

Foods like onion, garlic, radish, and leeks contain a natural antibiotic called "allicin," which increases immunity against many disease-producing organisms without any harmful effect to the body.

Foods like yeast, eggs, meat, seafood, wheat germ, cashew, non-fat milk, etc. are rich in minerals such as Zn and are preventives for thyroid disease. They also help to maintain a healthy weight.

Foods like oysters, shellfish, whole grains, barley, brown rice, sunflower seeds, sweet potatoes, cereals, eggs, etc. are rich in vitamin E as well as minerals such as Zn. They improve fertility and sex drive in males and females. Similarly, the amino acid arginine is helpful in improving sperm count.

Foods like wheat germ, oat meal, bran, onion, spinach, mushrooms, fish, chicken, skim milk, seafood, fruits and vegetable juices, asparagus, etc. contain good amounts of nucleic acids and the superoxide dismutase, which helps to slowdown aging for longer periods, making people look young.

Foods like soybeans, mushrooms, ginger, turmeric, fenugreek seeds, grape juice, berries, saledi (Baswellia serata), cruciferous vegetables, pomegranate, carrot, sesame seeds, oil or capsules of shark cartilage, etc. help to prevent and cure osteoarthritis.

Foods like fish oil, liver oil, soybean oil, canola oil, flaxseed oil, etc. are rich in omaga-3 fatty acids, which lower cholesterol and triglycerides in blood.

Foods like caraway, dill, ginger, yeast, raisins, cantaloupe, cereals, legumes, nuts, citrus fruits, tomato, citrus, medicago, etc. contain vitamin B1, B2, B9, B6, C and glycine, which improve gastrointestinal and gastric hyperacidity problems.

Foods like milk, cheese, meat, fish, dried dates, peanut, sesame, and banana are rich in protein while almonds, soybeans, etc. are rich in amino acids like phenylalanine, tryptophan, and tyrosine along with vitamin B1 and B9, which can act as antidepressants. Minerals like Ca, Mn and Zn also help to alleviate depression.

Foods like tea, kelp, salt, seafood, olives, milk and milk products, nuts, beans, broccoli, eggs, etc. are rich in minerals like Ca, P, Fl, I, Cl, etc., which contribute to strong teeth and gums. As a result, conditions like periodontitis, bleeding gums, tooth decay, tooth loss, etc. are alleviated.

Foods like papaya, carrot, mango, orange, cantaloupe, milk and milk products, eggs, green vegetables, fish, yeast, etc. are rich in vitamin A and B2, which can prevent eye problems.

Foods like grain cereals, legumes, milk and milk products, yeast, meat, fish, eggs, the leaves of Indian licorice, etc. contain vitamin B2 and B6, which help to alleviate mouth sores and cracks.

Foods like grain cereals, legumes, nuts, table salt, cheese, butter, yeast, eggs, meats, fish, sunshine, etc. are rich in vitamins B1, B6, B7, D as well as minerals like chlorine and sodium, which help to relieve muscle cramps.

Foods like cereals, beans, milk and milk products, yeast, nuts, green vegetables, citrus fruits, banana, cantaloupe, eggs, fish, meat, etc. are rich in vitamin B complex as well as minerals like potassium and calcium, which help to alleviate insomnia (Sleeplessness).

Foods like cereals, bran, corn, cruciferous vegetables, apple, garlic, carrot, beet, grapefruits, cantaloupe, fenugreek seeds, and onion contain good amounts of cellulose and hemicelluloses, which make for smooth functioning of the large intestine.

Foods like oatmeal, beans, cruciferous vegetables, citrus fruits, pears, strawberry, etc. are rich in gum, pectin, and lignin, which bind the bile acids and prevent the absorption of fat in the stomach and small intestine, lowering cholesterol and blood sugar levels.

Foods like onion, garlic, citrus fruits, tomato, cantaloupe, banana, dates, figs, avocado, potatoes, nuts, yeast, green vegetables are rich in vitamin E, B12, B3, choline, omega-3 fatty acids, as well as minerals like potassium, chromium, magnesium, which can lower blood pressure.

Foods like apples, grapes, raisins, etc. contain boron, which can retard bone loss in women after menopause as well as help to keep estrogen in the blood longer. In combination with Ca, Mg, and Vitamin D, boron also helps to prevent osteoporosis.

Foods like milk, cheese, yeast, green vegetables, meat, eggs, fish, cereals, and legumes are rich in vitamin B2 and B6, which help to eliminate lesions or sores of the mouth, lips, and tongue.

Foods like wheat germ, yeast, meat, eggs, nuts, soybeans, legumes, and green-leaf vegetables, contain vitamin B-choline, manganese, lipotropic, and phenylalanine, which help to improve memory in old age.

Foods like whole wheat, peanuts, dates, figs, meat, eggs, fish, avocado, etc. contain vitamin B3 (niacin), which is essential for the synthesis of the male sex hormone testosterone, and the female sex hormones progesterone and estrogen, as well as cortisone, thyroxin, and insulin. They can also reduce blood pressure, cholesterol, and triglycerides.

Foods like whole wheat, rice, beans, yeast, meat, eggs, avocado, carrot, green leafy vegetables, cantaloupe, etc. contain PABA (Paramine benzoic acid) and folic acid, which can return gray hair to its natural color.

Foods like yellow and orange fruits or vegetables like carrots, pumpkins, sweet potatoes, cantaloupe, etc. contain beta-carotene, which prevents heart diseases and many types of cancers.

Foods like milk and milk products, soybeans, peanuts, walnuts, sunflower seeds, beans, kale, broccoli, bananas, almonds, etc. contain minerals like magnesium, manganese, boron, calcium and vitamin D, which can prevent osteoporosis.

Foods like milk, cheese, meat, fish, bananas, dried dates, peanuts, and other protein-rich foods contain sulfur amino acid tryptophan, which induces natural sleep. When conventional pain killers are not working, then DLPA (D-phenylalanine) gives good results without any toxic or side effects.

Foods like eggs have a perfect protein component as compared to other foods. They also contain lecithin, which assimilates fat and raises the HDL level in blood.

XI. HOW NUTRIENTS ARE RETAINED IN FOODS

MOST FOODS CONTAIN some nutrients in various amounts. However, all these nutrients may not be available at the time of eating because loss of nutrients occurs during the transport, processing, storage, or cooking of the food. So it is essential to learn how we can retain the nutrients in foods by avoiding these losses.

- A grinding machine should generate minimum heat at the time of milling grain cereals, legumes, and other food grains into flour. This helps to retain more nutrients.
- Food materials should be stored in dry, cold places, so that losses due to oxidation and pest damage are avoided.
- Steam-cooked foods retain more nutrients than fried, water cooked, or roasted foods.
- Cooking foods in stainless steel, glass, or enamel cookware helps to retain more nutrients than cooking in copper, or brass.
- Less cooking with water and short cooking times help to retain more nutrients in foods.

- Milk in glass containers exposed to light will lose vitamin A, B2, and D. Milk should be stored away from light.
- After you've purchased vegetables and fruits at the market, they should be thoroughly washed with clean water at home and stored in the refrigerator till further use. This will help to retain more of their nutrients.
- Vegetables and fruits should be cut with a sharp knife to avoid the loss of nutrients. Cutting with a blunt knife causes the loss of vitamins due to bruising.
- Green salad should be prepared just before its use to avoid the loss of nutrients.
- The roasting of food until it turns brown or black causes the loss of many nutrients.
- Peanut, sesame, canola, and olive oils are suitable for frequent frying as well as for long periods of storage as compared to sunflower, safflower, and corn oils.
- The green and immature seeds of legumes like peas, pigeon peas, beans, lentils, black-eyed peas, etc. retain more nutrients as compared to the dried and matured seeds. This is because green seeds contain more nutrients than dried. They also are more digestible.
- Steam-cooked, green and immature kernels of maize retain more nutrients as compared to roasted or baked kernels.
- Brown rice contains more nutrients than white and polished rice.
- Generally, sprouted wheat and legumes contain more nutrients and are more digestible than unsprouted.
- Bread and other food products prepared from whole-wheat flour contain more nutrients and are better digestible than food preparations made from the more highly processed "Maida" flour.

XII. NUTRIENTS AND FOODS FOR SPECIFIC HEALTH PROBLEMS

Disease or Disorder	Nutrients Suggested	Foods Suggested
Appetite loss	Protein, Vitamin A, B1, B7, C, P, S, Zn	Cereals, legumes, nuts, milk and milk products, yeast, eggs, fish, SFS, green/yellow vegetables, citrus fruits
Alzheimer memory loss	B1, Choline	Cereals, dry legumes, nuts, yeast, meat, potatoes
Acne	Multiple vitamin, B-carotene	Grain cereals, nuts, green-leafy vegetables, soybeans, eggs
Arthritis	Vitamin C, B3, B5, B12, Cu	Grain cereals and legumes, yeast, meat, eggs, fish, citrus fruits
Asthma	Vitamin C, B2, B5, B6, E	Green/yellow vegetables, yeast, milk, meat, eggs, nuts, citrus fruits
Bluish, purplish, or colorless bruising	Vitamin C, Bioflavonoids	Citrus fruits, peas, berries, cabbage, tomatoes, peppers
Blood pressure	Vitamin E, B3, Choline, K, Ca, Mg, Cl, Omega-3, FA	Garlic, onions, kelp, green vegetables, yeast, grain cereals and legumes, soybean oil, flax oil, canola oil, fish oils

Bad breath	B3, Acidophilus, Zn	Grain cereals and legumes, dill
Baldness (hair loss)	Vitamin C, Choline, B7, Inositol, Cysteine, B9, Ca, Mg, Cl	Grain cereals, beans, nuts, yeast, raisins, meat, citrus fruits, green vegetables, potatoes, tomatoes, cantaloupe
Cholesterol	Vitamin B, Methionine	Peanuts, raisins, yeast, cantaloupe, grapefruit, cabbage
Bleeding gums	Vitamin C, complex, K, Bio-flavonoids rutin and hesperidin	Orange, lemon, lime, yogurt, kelp, soybean oil
Bronchitis	Vitamin C, E, BC, acidophilus	Citrus fruits, green-yellow vegetables, nuts
Diarrhea	Vit.B3, K, L-acid-ophilus	Yogurt, alfalfa, kelp, carrots, grain, cereals and legumes, yeast, peanuts, sunflower seeds, soybean oil, avocados, green vegetables
Dizziness	Vitamin B2, B3, E, Mn	Milk, cheese, yeast, nuts, peas, beets, meat, eggs, fish, green vegetables,
Diabetes	Vitamin B6, Gum pectin, glutathi-one, K, Cr, Zn	Cabbage, cauliflower, carrots, beans, oatmeal, citrus, bitter gourd, plums
Eczema	Vitamin A (Carot-ene), B-complex, Inositol, Cu, I	Grain cereals and legumes, nuts, milk and milk products, green/yellow vegetables
Tinnitus	Vitamin B3, E, Mu, K, Zn	Grain cereals and legumes, nuts, SFS*, peas, eggs, green vege-tables, citrus fruits, beets
Eye problems; night-blind-ness, blood shot, inflam-mation	Vitamin A (C), B2, C, E	Green/yellow vegetables, fruits, nuts, peas, eggs, SFS, butter, cream, yeast, fish, meat
Fatigue, weakness, inactivity, dullness	Protein, Carbohy-drates, Vitamin A, B, C, D, Zn, Fe, I	Grain cereals and legumes, milk and milk products, yeast, beans, eggs, meat, fish, green/yellow vegetables, citrus fruits, seafoods

Gastro-intestinal disorders, gastritis, indigestion, gastric problems, hyperacidity	Vitamin B1, B2, B5, B9, C, Cl	Grain cereals and legumes, nuts, milk and milk products, yeast, eggs, fish, citrus fruits, green/yellow vegetables, tomatoes, cantaloupe, onion, garlic
Heart issues like palpitations, heart attacks, blood pressure, cholesterol	Vitamin B3, B12, E	Grain cereals and legumes, nuts, SFS, peas, meat, fish, eggs, green vegetables, citrus fruits
Hair problems, Dandruff	Vitamin B6, B12, B12, Selenium	Grain cereals and legumes, SFS, nuts, milk and milk products, meat, eggs, fish, yeast, onions, tomatoes
Graying hair	Vitamin A, Pyro-benzoic acid, iodine	Milk and milk products, unsaturated oils, nuts, bran, yeast, seafood, raisins, carrots, cantaloupe
Hair loss	Vitamin B7, B9, C, Inositol, Chlorine	Grain cereals, nuts, yeast, table salt, brans, cabbage, potatoes, tomatoes, green-leafy vegetables
Insomnia	B-complex, B6, K, Ca, Tryptophan	Yeast, cereals, nuts, beans, milk and milk products, meat, eggs, fish, fruits, vegetables canta-loupe, raisins
Itching	Vitamin B5, C, E, E-Cyclam, Iodine, Antihistamine	Cereals and legumes, yeast, meat, fish, seafoods, citrus fruits
Loss of sense of smell	Vitamin A, Zn	Green-yellow vegetables, fish, eggs, butter, grain cereals, SFS
Memory loss	Vitamin B1, Choline, L-gluta-mine	Grain cereals and legumes, nuts, yeast, potatoes, soybeans, olives
Menstrual problems	Vitamin B6, B12, Mg, Ca	Grain cereals and legumes, meat, fish, eggs, nuts, green-leafy vegetables

Menopause	Vitamin E, B-complex, Ca, Mg, Se	Cereals, brans, milk, nuts, meat, eggs, yeast, broccoli, onion, tomatoes, green vegetables
Mouth sores	Vitamin B2, B6	Grain cereals and legumes, milk and milk products, yeast, meat, eggs, fish
Muscle cramps, night cramps	Vitamin B1, B6, B3, B7, D, Cl, Ca, Mg	Grain cereals and legumes, nuts, yeast, eggs, meat, fish, potatoes, butter, sunshine
Nose bleeds	Vitamin C, K, Bioflavonoids	Citrus fruits, tomatoes, potatoes, cabbage, kelp, green peppers, yogurt
Skin problems, acne	Vitamin A, (BC), E, B-Complex, Zn	Soybean oil, fish oil, green-yellow vegetables, butter, cream, yeast, eggs, fish, beans, cantaloupe, raisins
Dermatitis	Vitamin B2, B3, B6, B7, E, BC, Zn	Grain cereals and legumes, milk, cheese, yeast, meat, eggs, fish
Eczema	Vitamin A (BC), E, B-complex, Cu, I	Grain cereals and legumes, nuts, milk products, yeast, green-yellow vegetables, butter, eggs, fish, seafoods
Slow healing wounds, fractures	Vitamin E, Zn	Citrus fruits, berries, tomatoes, potatoes, cabbage, nuts, SFS, grain cereals, vegetables
Softening of bones and teeth	Vitamin D, Ca, Mg	Grain cereals and legumes, milk and milk products, nuts, meat, eggs, fish, green leafy vegetables, sunshine
Prostate problems	Zn	Soybean, SFS, grain cereals, vegetables, nuts

*SFS (Sunflower Seeds)

1) The production of growth hormone from the pituitary gland is reduced with age. As a result, our immunity against diseases also decreases. This can be reversed by taking in more nutrients like amino acids, especially arginine,

ornithine, and cystine along with vitamins A, C, E, etc. and minerals like Zinc and selenium.

2) Vitamin K prevents internal bleeding and hemorrhages and promotes blood clotting. It reduces excessive menstrual flow. It's available from foods like green vegetables, spinach, yogurt, safflower oil, soybean oil, kelp, fish liver oil, etc.

3) Senior citizens require more nutrients like Vitamin A, B-9, B-12, C, D, E, and K as well as minerals like calcium, magnesium, and iron for maintaining good health. These are available from foods like grain cereals, legumes, nuts, citrus fruits, papaya, apple, tomato, milk, green leafy vegetables, etc.

4) Yeast contains most of the Vitamin B complex, fifteen amino acids, more than fourteen minerals, and seventeen vitamins, excluding A, C, and E. It is a complete food. A tablespoon of yeast taken in liquid restores energy very quickly.

XIII. VITAMIN FUNCTION AND FOOD SOURCES

Name of Vitamin	Important Health Function	Availability from Foods
Vitamin-A Retinol (Animal Source) B-Carotene (Plant source)	Eyes, skin, hair, teeth, gums, bones, heart, immunity	Papaya, guava, mango, cantaloupe, kiwi, lychee, orange, peach, avocado, carrot, spinach, milk and milk products, eggs, fish, meat
Vitamin B-complex		
Vitamin B1 (Thymine)	Nerves, muscles, heart, mental attitude, appetite, paralysis	Cereals, nuts, beans, milk, vegetables, meat, spotato*, yeast
Vitamin B2 (Riboflavin)	Skin, nails, hair, eyes, reproduction, prostate, and sores of the mouth, lips, and tongue	Milk, cheese, sesame, soybean, spinach, meat, eggs, fish, yeast
Vitamin B3 (Niacin)	Blood pressure, cholesterol, bad breath, triglycerides, sex hormones, gastrointestinal	Whole grains, yeast, peanut, peas, avocado, dates, figs, meat, eggs, fish
Vitamin B5 (Pantothenic acid)	Wound healing, RBC*, nervous system, antibody production	Whole grains, yeast, nuts, meat, lentil, sesame, avocado, green vegetables, mushrooms, potatoes, SFS*

Vitamin B6 (Pyridoxine)	Production of RBC, nucleic acid and antibodies, diuretic, nervousness	Whole wheat, beans, nuts, SFS, fish, meat, eggs, yeast, banana, avocado, cabbage, spinach, sweet potato, potato
Vitamin B7 (Biotin)	Prevents gray hair and baldness, skin diseases, muscle pain, promotes production of breast milk	Soybean, milk, nuts, yogurt, yeast, meat, eggs, banana, carrot, broccoli, tomato
Vitamin B9 (Folic acid)	Production of nucleic acids, RBC, prevents birth defects, prevents gray hair,	Cereals, sesame, corn, yeast, cantaloupe, avocado, carrot, beans, peas, green vegetables, orange, SFS, papaya
Vitamin B12 (Cobalamin)	Memory, muscles, RBC, synthesis, growth and appetite in children, nerves	Milk, cheese, yogurt, eggs, fish, meat
Vitamin C (Ascorbic acid)	Bruising, common cold, gum disease, depression, scurvy	Citrus fruits, guava, berries, pineapple, grape, spinach, broccoli, peas, mango, papaya, tomato, cauliflower
Vitamin D (7-Dhydro cholesterol)	Strong bone and teeth, blood pressure, depression, tooth decay, rickets	Milk and milk products, fish, liver oil, mushroom, eggs, oranges, sunlight
Vitamin E (Tocopherol)	Skin, hair, blood pressure, antiaging, sex hormones, anticoagulant	Almond, peanut, whole grains, soybean, eggs, green vegetables, SFS, kiwi, mango, avocado
Vitamin K (Menadione)	Blood clotting, prevents bleeding, hemorrhage, excessive menstrual flow, heart disease, cancer, diabetes	Cabbage, carrot, cucumber, kale, onion, soybean oil, fish, liver oil, spinach, lettuce, yogurt, avocado, broccoli

Note: SFS (Sunflower Seeds), Spotato (Sweet potato), RBC (Red blood cell)

BIBLIOGRAPHY

Adams, Ruth and Frank Murray. *Minerals: Kill or Cure.* New York: Larchmont Books, 1976.

Bailey, Hubert. *Vitamin E: Your Key to a Healthy Heart.* New York: ARC Books, 1964, 1966

Bernardini, E. 1985. "Oilseeds, Oil and Fats." Vol. I *Intersperma*, Roma.

Borsaak, Henry. *Vitamins: What They Are and How They Can Benefit You.* New York: Pyramid Books, 1971

"Buying Beef." *Consumer Reports* 39 (September 1974)

Clark, Linda. *The Best of Linda Clark.* New Canaan, CT: Keats Publishing Co., 1976.

--- *Know Your Nutrition.* New Canaan, CT: Keats Publishing Co., 1973

---*Secrets of Health and Beauty.* New York: Jove Publication, 1977.

Cooper, Kenneth H. M.D. *Overcoming Hypertension.* New York: Bantam Books, 1990

Ebon, Martin. *Which Vitamins Do You Need?* New York: Bantam Books, 1974.

Flynn, Margaret A. "The Cholesterol Controversy." *Journal of the American Pharmacy* NS18 (May 1978).

"Food Facts Talk Back. *"Journal of the American Dietetic Association*, 1977

Fredericks Carlton. *Look Younger Feel Healthier.* New York: Grosset and Dunlap, 1977

Goodhart, Robert S., and Maurice E. Shills. *Modern Nutrition in Health and Disease.* 5th ed. Philadelphia: Lea and Fibger, 1973.

Journal of Applied Nutrition. International College of Applied Nutrition, La Habra, CA, 1974-76.

Kordel, L. *Health Through Nutrition.* New York: Mac-Fadden-Bartell, 1971.

Murphy, D.J. 1993. *Designer Oil Crops Breeding, Processing and Biotechnology.* VCH Publishers, New York.

Nagaraj, G. 1990. "Biochemical Quality of Oilseeds," Journal of Oilseeds Research. 7:47-55.

Nagaraj, G. 1995. "Quality and Utility of Oilseeds." Directorate of Oilseeds Research, Hyderabad.

"Nutritional Information Resources for the Whole Family." National Nutrition Education Clearing House. 1978.

Pritikin, Nathan. *The Pritikin Permanent Weight-Loss Manual.* New York: Grosset & Dunlap, 1981.

Rodale, J.I. *The Complete Book of Minerals for Health*. 4th ed. Emmaus, PA: Rodale Books, 1976.

Rosenberg, Harold, and A.N. Feldzaman. *Doctor's Book of Vitamin Therapy: Megavitamins for Health*. New York: Putnam's, 1974.

Salunkhe, D.K. et al. *World Oilseeds - Chemistry, Technology and Utilization*. Avi Book, Van Nostrand Reinhold, New York. 1991

Smith, Lendon, M.D. *Feed Yourself Right*. New York: McGraw Hill, 1983.

United National, Food and Agriculture Organization. Calorie Requirements, 1957, 1972.

U.S. Department of Agriculture. "Amino Acid Content of Food" by M.L. Orr and B.K. Watt, 1957: rev. 1968.

U.S. Department of Agriculture. "Consumer and Food Ecosition of Foods: Raw, Processed, Prepared," by Bernice K. Watt and Annabel. L. Merrill, 1975.

Carlson, Wade. *Vitamin E: The Rejuvenation Vitamin*. New York: Award Books, 1970.

"Which Cereals are Most Nutritious?" *Consumer Reports* 40 (February 1975).

Winter, Ruth. *A Consumer's Dictionary of Food Additives*. New York: Crown, 1973.